THIS BOOK BELONGS TO:

NAME	
ADDRESS	
PHONE #	
EMAIL	

Copyright © Teresa Rother
All rights reserved. No part of this publication may be reproduced, distributed, or transmitted in any form or by any means, including photocopy, recording, or other electronic or mechanical methods.

DEDICATION

This Juicing Recipe Book is dedicated to all the people who want to keep track of their favorite juicing and smoothie recipes.

You are my inspiration for producing this book and I'm honored to be a part of your record-keeping and organization.

HOW TO USE THIS BOOK

This Juicing Book will help you by accurately recording recipes in an easy to use format.

Here are examples of information for you to fill in and write the details of your book.

Fill in the following information:

1. Shopping List - For writing down frequently used ingredients.

2. Prep Time - Record the time it takes to make the recipe.

3. Juicing Time - Record time spent juicing.

4. Number of Ounces - Record the measurement.

5. Number Of Servings - List number of servings for recipe.

6. Juicing Is For - Checklist for breakfast, lunch, dinner, or healing.

7. Ingredients - Write down a list of ingredients.

8. How To Prepare - Write down the process and preparation steps for your recipe.

9. How I Felt - Jot down the effects on your body and health after drinking the juice.

10. My Results - Checklist for tracking improvements in mood, energy, focus, and weight loss.

11. Juice Rating - Rate the recipe using a number system 1 through 10.

INGREDIENT LIST

JUICE RECIPE

PREP TIME		# OF OUNCES	
JUICING TIME		# OF SERVINGS	

THIS JUICE IS FOR:

○ BREAKFAST   ○ LUNCH   ○ DINNER   ○ HEALING

INGREDIENTS

_____
_____
_____
_____
_____
_____
_____
_____
_____

HOW TO PREPARE

_____
_____
_____
_____

HOW I FELT AFTER JUICING

_____
_____

MY RESULTS	○ IMPROVED MOOD ○ IMPROVED ENERGY ○ IMPROVED FOCUS ○ WEIGHTLOSS
MY RATING FOR THIS JUICE RECIPE	○1 ○2 ○3 ○4 ○5 ○6 ○7 ○8 ○9 ○10

JUICE RECIPE

PREP TIME		# OF OUNCES	
JUICING TIME		# OF SERVINGS	

THIS JUICE IS FOR:

○ BREAKFAST   ○ LUNCH   ○ DINNER   ○ HEALING

INGREDIENTS

_____
_____
_____
_____
_____
_____
_____
_____

HOW TO PREPARE

_____
_____
_____
_____

HOW I FELT AFTER JUICING

_____
_____
_____

MY RESULTS	○ IMPROVED MOOD ○ IMPROVED ENERGY ○ IMPROVED FOCUS ○ WEIGHTLOSS
MY RATING FOR THIS JUICE RECIPE	○1 ○2 ○3 ○4 ○5 ○6 ○7 ○8 ○9 ○10

JUICE RECIPE

PREP TIME		# OF OUNCES	
JUICING TIME		# OF SERVINGS	

THIS JUICE IS FOR:

○ BREAKFAST   ○ LUNCH   ○ DINNER   ○ HEALING

INGREDIENTS

HOW TO PREPARE

HOW I FELT AFTER JUICING

MY RESULTS	○ IMPROVED MOOD ○ IMPROVED ENERGY ○ IMPROVED FOCUS ○ WEIGHTLOSS
MY RATING FOR THIS JUICE RECIPE	○1 ○2 ○3 ○4 ○5 ○6 ○7 ○8 ○9 ○10

JUICE RECIPE

PREP TIME		# OF OUNCES	
JUICING TIME		# OF SERVINGS	

THIS JUICE IS FOR:

○ BREAKFAST　　○ LUNCH　　○ DINNER　　○ HEALING

INGREDIENTS

_____
_____
_____
_____
_____
_____
_____
_____

HOW TO PREPARE

_____
_____
_____
_____

HOW I FELT AFTER JUICING

_____
_____
_____

MY RESULTS	○ IMPROVED MOOD　○ IMPROVED ENERGY　○ IMPROVED FOCUS　○ WEIGHTLOSS
MY RATING FOR THIS JUICE RECIPE	○1　○2　○3　○4　○5　○6　○7　○8　○9　○10

JUICE RECIPE

PREP TIME		# OF OUNCES	
JUICING TIME		# OF SERVINGS	

THIS JUICE IS FOR:

○ BREAKFAST	○ LUNCH	○ DINNER	○ HEALING

INGREDIENTS

_____
_____
_____
_____
_____
_____
_____
_____
_____
_____

HOW TO PREPARE

_____
_____
_____
_____

HOW I FELT AFTER JUICING

_____
_____
_____

MY RESULTS	○ IMPROVED MOOD ○ IMPROVED ENERGY ○ IMPROVED FOCUS ○ WEIGHTLOSS
MY RATING FOR THIS JUICE RECIPE	○1 ○2 ○3 ○4 ○5 ○6 ○7 ○8 ○9 ○10

JUICE RECIPE

PREP TIME		# OF OUNCES	
JUICING TIME		# OF SERVINGS	

THIS JUICE IS FOR:

○ BREAKFAST ○ LUNCH ○ DINNER ○ HEALING

INGREDIENTS

_____
_____
_____
_____
_____
_____
_____
_____
_____

HOW TO PREPARE

_____
_____
_____
_____

HOW I FELT AFTER JUICING

_____
_____

MY RESULTS	○ IMPROVED MOOD ○ IMPROVED ENERGY ○ IMPROVED FOCUS ○ WEIGHTLOSS
MY RATING FOR THIS JUICE RECIPE	○1 ○2 ○3 ○4 ○5 ○6 ○7 ○8 ○9 ○10

JUICE RECIPE

PREP TIME		# OF OUNCES	
JUICING TIME		# OF SERVINGS	

THIS JUICE IS FOR:

○ BREAKFAST	○ LUNCH	○ DINNER	○ HEALING

INGREDIENTS

HOW TO PREPARE

HOW I FELT AFTER JUICING

MY RESULTS	○ IMPROVED MOOD ○ IMPROVED ENERGY ○ IMPROVED FOCUS ○ WEIGHTLOSS
MY RATING FOR THIS JUICE RECIPE	○ 1 ○ 2 ○ 3 ○ 4 ○ 5 ○ 6 ○ 7 ○ 8 ○ 9 ○ 10

JUICE RECIPE

PREP TIME		# OF OUNCES	
JUICING TIME		# OF SERVINGS	

THIS JUICE IS FOR:

| ○ BREAKFAST | ○ LUNCH | ○ DINNER | ○ HEALING |

INGREDIENTS

_____
_____
_____
_____
_____
_____
_____
_____
_____

HOW TO PREPARE

_____
_____
_____
_____
_____

HOW I FELT AFTER JUICING

_____
_____

MY RESULTS	○ IMPROVED MOOD ○ IMPROVED ENERGY ○ IMPROVED FOCUS ○ WEIGHTLOSS
MY RATING FOR THIS JUICE RECIPE	○1 ○2 ○3 ○4 ○5 ○6 ○7 ○8 ○9 ○10

JUICE RECIPE

PREP TIME		# OF OUNCES	
JUICING TIME		# OF SERVINGS	

THIS JUICE IS FOR:

○ BREAKFAST	○ LUNCH	○ DINNER	○ HEALING

INGREDIENTS

_____
_____
_____
_____
_____
_____
_____
_____
_____
_____

HOW TO PREPARE

_____
_____
_____
_____

HOW I FELT AFTER JUICING

_____
_____

MY RESULTS	○ IMPROVED MOOD ○ IMPROVED ENERGY ○ IMPROVED FOCUS ○ WEIGHTLOSS
MY RATING FOR THIS JUICE RECIPE	○1 ○2 ○3 ○4 ○5 ○6 ○7 ○8 ○9 ○10

JUICE RECIPE

PREP TIME		# OF OUNCES	
JUICING TIME		# OF SERVINGS	

THIS JUICE IS FOR:

○ BREAKFAST	○ LUNCH	○ DINNER	○ HEALING

INGREDIENTS

_____

_____

_____

_____

_____

_____

_____

_____

HOW TO PREPARE

_____

_____

_____

_____

HOW I FELT AFTER JUICING

_____

_____

MY RESULTS	○ IMPROVED MOOD ○ IMPROVED ENERGY ○ IMPROVED FOCUS ○ WEIGHTLOSS
MY RATING FOR THIS JUICE RECIPE	○1 ○2 ○3 ○4 ○5 ○6 ○7 ○8 ○9 ○10

JUICE RECIPE

PREP TIME		# OF OUNCES	
JUICING TIME		# OF SERVINGS	

THIS JUICE IS FOR:

○ BREAKFAST	○ LUNCH	○ DINNER	○ HEALING

INGREDIENTS

_____
_____
_____
_____
_____
_____
_____
_____
_____
_____

HOW TO PREPARE

_____
_____
_____
_____

HOW I FELT AFTER JUICING

_____
_____

MY RESULTS	○ IMPROVED MOOD ○ IMPROVED ENERGY ○ IMPROVED FOCUS ○ WEIGHTLOSS
MY RATING FOR THIS JUICE RECIPE	○1 ○2 ○3 ○4 ○5 ○6 ○7 ○8 ○9 ○10

JUICE RECIPE

PREP TIME		# OF OUNCES	
JUICING TIME		# OF SERVINGS	

THIS JUICE IS FOR:

○ BREAKFAST ○ LUNCH ○ DINNER ○ HEALING

INGREDIENTS

_____
_____
_____
_____
_____
_____
_____
_____
_____

HOW TO PREPARE

_____
_____
_____
_____

HOW I FELT AFTER JUICING

_____
_____
_____

MY RESULTS	○ IMPROVED MOOD ○ IMPROVED ENERGY ○ IMPROVED FOCUS ○ WEIGHTLOSS
MY RATING FOR THIS JUICE RECIPE	○ 1 ○ 2 ○ 3 ○ 4 ○ 5 ○ 6 ○ 7 ○ 8 ○ 9 ○ 10

JUICE RECIPE

PREP TIME		# OF OUNCES	
JUICING TIME		# OF SERVINGS	

THIS JUICE IS FOR:

○ BREAKFAST	○ LUNCH	○ DINNER	○ HEALING

INGREDIENTS

HOW TO PREPARE

HOW I FELT AFTER JUICING

MY RESULTS	○ IMPROVED MOOD ○ IMPROVED ENERGY ○ IMPROVED FOCUS ○ WEIGHTLOSS
MY RATING FOR THIS JUICE RECIPE	○1 ○2 ○3 ○4 ○5 ○6 ○7 ○8 ○9 ○10

JUICE RECIPE

PREP TIME		# OF OUNCES	
JUICING TIME		# OF SERVINGS	

THIS JUICE IS FOR:

○ BREAKFAST	○ LUNCH	○ DINNER	○ HEALING

INGREDIENTS

_____
_____
_____
_____
_____
_____
_____
_____

HOW TO PREPARE

_____
_____
_____
_____

HOW I FELT AFTER JUICING

_____
_____
_____

MY RESULTS	○ IMPROVED MOOD ○ IMPROVED ENERGY ○ IMPROVED FOCUS ○ WEIGHTLOSS
MY RATING FOR THIS JUICE RECIPE	○1 ○2 ○3 ○4 ○5 ○6 ○7 ○8 ○9 ○10

JUICE RECIPE

PREP TIME		# OF OUNCES	
JUICING TIME		# OF SERVINGS	

THIS JUICE IS FOR:

○ BREAKFAST　　○ LUNCH　　○ DINNER　　○ HEALING

INGREDIENTS

_____
_____
_____
_____
_____
_____
_____
_____
_____
_____

HOW TO PREPARE

_____
_____
_____
_____

HOW I FELT AFTER JUICING

_____
_____

MY RESULTS	○ IMPROVED MOOD　○ IMPROVED ENERGY　○ IMPROVED FOCUS　○ WEIGHTLOSS
MY RATING FOR THIS JUICE RECIPE	○1　○2　○3　○4　○5　○6　○7　○8　○9　○10

JUICE RECIPE

PREP TIME		# OF OUNCES	
JUICING TIME		# OF SERVINGS	

THIS JUICE IS FOR:

| ○ BREAKFAST | ○ LUNCH | ○ DINNER | ○ HEALING |

INGREDIENTS

_____
_____
_____
_____
_____
_____
_____
_____

HOW TO PREPARE

_____
_____
_____
_____

HOW I FELT AFTER JUICING

_____
_____

| MY RESULTS | ○ IMPROVED MOOD ○ IMPROVED ENERGY ○ IMPROVED FOCUS ○ WEIGHTLOSS |
| MY RATING FOR THIS JUICE RECIPE | ○1 ○2 ○3 ○4 ○5 ○6 ○7 ○8 ○9 ○10 |

JUICE RECIPE

PREP TIME		# OF OUNCES	
JUICING TIME		# OF SERVINGS	

THIS JUICE IS FOR:

○ BREAKFAST	○ LUNCH	○ DINNER	○ HEALING

INGREDIENTS

HOW TO PREPARE

HOW I FELT AFTER JUICING

MY RESULTS	○ IMPROVED MOOD ○ IMPROVED ENERGY ○ IMPROVED FOCUS ○ WEIGHTLOSS
MY RATING FOR THIS JUICE RECIPE	○1 ○2 ○3 ○4 ○5 ○6 ○7 ○8 ○9 ○10

JUICE RECIPE

PREP TIME		# OF OUNCES	
JUICING TIME		# OF SERVINGS	

THIS JUICE IS FOR:

○ BREAKFAST	○ LUNCH	○ DINNER	○ HEALING

INGREDIENTS

_____
_____
_____
_____
_____
_____
_____
_____
_____

HOW TO PREPARE

_____
_____
_____
_____

HOW I FELT AFTER JUICING

_____
_____

MY RESULTS	○ IMPROVED MOOD ○ IMPROVED ENERGY ○ IMPROVED FOCUS ○ WEIGHTLOSS
MY RATING FOR THIS JUICE RECIPE	○1 ○2 ○3 ○4 ○5 ○6 ○7 ○8 ○9 ○10

JUICE RECIPE

PREP TIME		# OF OUNCES	
JUICING TIME		# OF SERVINGS	

THIS JUICE IS FOR:

○ BREAKFAST   ○ LUNCH   ○ DINNER   ○ HEALING

INGREDIENTS

_____
_____
_____
_____
_____
_____
_____
_____
_____
_____

HOW TO PREPARE

_____
_____
_____
_____

HOW I FELT AFTER JUICING

_____
_____
_____

MY RESULTS	○ IMPROVED MOOD ○ IMPROVED ENERGY ○ IMPROVED FOCUS ○ WEIGHTLOSS
MY RATING FOR THIS JUICE RECIPE	○ 1 ○ 2 ○ 3 ○ 4 ○ 5 ○ 6 ○ 7 ○ 8 ○ 9 ○ 10

JUICE RECIPE

PREP TIME		# OF OUNCES	
JUICING TIME		# OF SERVINGS	

THIS JUICE IS FOR:

| ○ BREAKFAST | ○ LUNCH | ○ DINNER | ○ HEALING |

INGREDIENTS

_____
_____
_____
_____
_____
_____
_____
_____

HOW TO PREPARE

_____
_____
_____
_____

HOW I FELT AFTER JUICING

_____
_____

MY RESULTS	○ IMPROVED MOOD ○ IMPROVED ENERGY ○ IMPROVED FOCUS ○ WEIGHTLOSS
MY RATING FOR THIS JUICE RECIPE	○ 1 ○ 2 ○ 3 ○ 4 ○ 5 ○ 6 ○ 7 ○ 8 ○ 9 ○ 10

JUICE RECIPE

PREP TIME		# OF OUNCES	
JUICING TIME		# OF SERVINGS	

THIS JUICE IS FOR:

○ BREAKFAST ○ LUNCH ○ DINNER ○ HEALING

INGREDIENTS

HOW TO PREPARE

HOW I FELT AFTER JUICING

MY RESULTS	○ IMPROVED MOOD ○ IMPROVED ENERGY ○ IMPROVED FOCUS ○ WEIGHTLOSS
MY RATING FOR THIS JUICE RECIPE	○1 ○2 ○3 ○4 ○5 ○6 ○7 ○8 ○9 ○10

JUICE RECIPE

PREP TIME		# OF OUNCES	
JUICING TIME		# OF SERVINGS	

THIS JUICE IS FOR:

○ BREAKFAST	○ LUNCH	○ DINNER	○ HEALING

INGREDIENTS

_____
_____
_____
_____
_____
_____
_____
_____

HOW TO PREPARE

_____
_____
_____
_____

HOW I FELT AFTER JUICING

_____
_____
_____

MY RESULTS	○ IMPROVED MOOD ○ IMPROVED ENERGY ○ IMPROVED FOCUS ○ WEIGHTLOSS
MY RATING FOR THIS JUICE RECIPE	○1 ○2 ○3 ○4 ○5 ○6 ○7 ○8 ○9 ○10

JUICE RECIPE

PREP TIME		# OF OUNCES	
JUICING TIME		# OF SERVINGS	

THIS JUICE IS FOR:

○ BREAKFAST	○ LUNCH	○ DINNER	○ HEALING

INGREDIENTS

_____
_____
_____
_____
_____
_____
_____
_____
_____

HOW TO PREPARE

_____
_____
_____
_____

HOW I FELT AFTER JUICING

_____
_____

MY RESULTS	○ IMPROVED MOOD ○ IMPROVED ENERGY ○ IMPROVED FOCUS ○ WEIGHTLOSS
MY RATING FOR THIS JUICE RECIPE	○1 ○2 ○3 ○4 ○5 ○6 ○7 ○8 ○9 ○10

JUICE RECIPE

PREP TIME		# OF OUNCES	
JUICING TIME		# OF SERVINGS	

THIS JUICE IS FOR:

○ BREAKFAST   ○ LUNCH   ○ DINNER   ○ HEALING

INGREDIENTS

_____
_____
_____
_____
_____
_____
_____
_____
_____
_____

HOW TO PREPARE

_____
_____
_____
_____

HOW I FELT AFTER JUICING

_____
_____

MY RESULTS	○ IMPROVED MOOD ○ IMPROVED ENERGY ○ IMPROVED FOCUS ○ WEIGHTLOSS
MY RATING FOR THIS JUICE RECIPE	○1 ○2 ○3 ○4 ○5 ○6 ○7 ○8 ○9 ○10

JUICE RECIPE

PREP TIME		# OF OUNCES	
JUICING TIME		# OF SERVINGS	

THIS JUICE IS FOR:

○ BREAKFAST ○ LUNCH ○ DINNER ○ HEALING

INGREDIENTS

_____
_____
_____
_____
_____
_____
_____
_____
_____

HOW TO PREPARE

_____
_____
_____
_____

HOW I FELT AFTER JUICING

_____
_____

MY RESULTS	○ IMPROVED MOOD ○ IMPROVED ENERGY ○ IMPROVED FOCUS ○ WEIGHTLOSS
MY RATING FOR THIS JUICE RECIPE	○1 ○2 ○3 ○4 ○5 ○6 ○7 ○8 ○9 ○10

JUICE RECIPE

PREP TIME		# OF OUNCES	
JUICING TIME		# OF SERVINGS	

THIS JUICE IS FOR:

○ BREAKFAST	○ LUNCH	○ DINNER	○ HEALING

INGREDIENTS

_____
_____
_____
_____
_____
_____
_____
_____

HOW TO PREPARE

_____
_____
_____
_____

HOW I FELT AFTER JUICING

_____
_____

MY RESULTS	○ IMPROVED MOOD ○ IMPROVED ENERGY ○ IMPROVED FOCUS ○ WEIGHTLOSS
MY RATING FOR THIS JUICE RECIPE	○1 ○2 ○3 ○4 ○5 ○6 ○7 ○8 ○9 ○10

JUICE RECIPE

PREP TIME		# OF OUNCES	
JUICING TIME		# OF SERVINGS	

THIS JUICE IS FOR:

○ BREAKFAST　　○ LUNCH　　○ DINNER　　○ HEALING

INGREDIENTS

HOW TO PREPARE

HOW I FELT AFTER JUICING

MY RESULTS	○ IMPROVED MOOD　○ IMPROVED ENERGY　○ IMPROVED FOCUS　○ WEIGHTLOSS
MY RATING FOR THIS JUICE RECIPE	○1　○2　○3　○4　○5　○6　○7　○8　○9　○10

JUICE RECIPE

PREP TIME		# OF OUNCES	
JUICING TIME		# OF SERVINGS	

THIS JUICE IS FOR:

○ BREAKFAST	○ LUNCH	○ DINNER	○ HEALING

INGREDIENTS

_____

_____

_____

_____

_____

_____

_____

_____

HOW TO PREPARE

_____

_____

_____

_____

HOW I FELT AFTER JUICING

_____

_____

_____

MY RESULTS	○ IMPROVED MOOD ○ IMPROVED ENERGY ○ IMPROVED FOCUS ○ WEIGHTLOSS
MY RATING FOR THIS JUICE RECIPE	○ 1 ○ 2 ○ 3 ○ 4 ○ 5 ○ 6 ○ 7 ○ 8 ○ 9 ○ 10

JUICE RECIPE

PREP TIME		# OF OUNCES	
JUICING TIME		# OF SERVINGS	

THIS JUICE IS FOR:

○ BREAKFAST   ○ LUNCH   ○ DINNER   ○ HEALING

INGREDIENTS

_____
_____
_____
_____
_____
_____
_____
_____
_____

HOW TO PREPARE

_____
_____
_____
_____

HOW I FELT AFTER JUICING

_____
_____

MY RESULTS	○ IMPROVED MOOD ○ IMPROVED ENERGY ○ IMPROVED FOCUS ○ WEIGHTLOSS
MY RATING FOR THIS JUICE RECIPE	○1 ○2 ○3 ○4 ○5 ○6 ○7 ○8 ○9 ○10

JUICE RECIPE

PREP TIME		# OF OUNCES	
JUICING TIME		# OF SERVINGS	

THIS JUICE IS FOR:

○ BREAKFAST ○ LUNCH ○ DINNER ○ HEALING

INGREDIENTS

_____
_____
_____
_____
_____
_____
_____
_____
_____

HOW TO PREPARE

_____
_____
_____
_____

HOW I FELT AFTER JUICING

_____
_____

MY RESULTS	○ IMPROVED MOOD ○ IMPROVED ENERGY ○ IMPROVED FOCUS ○ WEIGHTLOSS
MY RATING FOR THIS JUICE RECIPE	○1 ○2 ○3 ○4 ○5 ○6 ○7 ○8 ○9 ○10

JUICE RECIPE

PREP TIME		# OF OUNCES	
JUICING TIME		# OF SERVINGS	

THIS JUICE IS FOR:

○ BREAKFAST   ○ LUNCH   ○ DINNER   ○ HEALING

INGREDIENTS

_____
_____
_____
_____
_____
_____
_____
_____
_____

HOW TO PREPARE

_____
_____
_____
_____

HOW I FELT AFTER JUICING

_____
_____

MY RESULTS	○ IMPROVED MOOD ○ IMPROVED ENERGY ○ IMPROVED FOCUS ○ WEIGHTLOSS
MY RATING FOR THIS JUICE RECIPE	○1 ○2 ○3 ○4 ○5 ○6 ○7 ○8 ○9 ○10

JUICE RECIPE

PREP TIME		# OF OUNCES	
JUICING TIME		# OF SERVINGS	

THIS JUICE IS FOR:

○ BREAKFAST ○ LUNCH ○ DINNER ○ HEALING

INGREDIENTS

_____
_____
_____
_____
_____
_____
_____
_____

HOW TO PREPARE

_____
_____
_____
_____

HOW I FELT AFTER JUICING

_____
_____

MY RESULTS	○ IMPROVED MOOD ○ IMPROVED ENERGY ○ IMPROVED FOCUS ○ WEIGHTLOSS
MY RATING FOR THIS JUICE RECIPE	○1 ○2 ○3 ○4 ○5 ○6 ○7 ○8 ○9 ○10

JUICE RECIPE

PREP TIME		# OF OUNCES	
JUICING TIME		# OF SERVINGS	

THIS JUICE IS FOR:

○ BREAKFAST   ○ LUNCH   ○ DINNER   ○ HEALING

INGREDIENTS

HOW TO PREPARE

HOW I FELT AFTER JUICING

MY RESULTS	○ IMPROVED MOOD ○ IMPROVED ENERGY ○ IMPROVED FOCUS ○ WEIGHTLOSS
MY RATING FOR THIS JUICE RECIPE	○1 ○2 ○3 ○4 ○5 ○6 ○7 ○8 ○9 ○10

JUICE RECIPE

PREP TIME		# OF OUNCES	
JUICING TIME		# OF SERVINGS	

THIS JUICE IS FOR:

○ BREAKFAST ○ LUNCH ○ DINNER ○ HEALING

INGREDIENTS

_____
_____
_____
_____
_____
_____
_____
_____

HOW TO PREPARE

_____
_____
_____
_____

HOW I FELT AFTER JUICING

_____
_____
_____

MY RESULTS	○ IMPROVED MOOD ○ IMPROVED ENERGY ○ IMPROVED FOCUS ○ WEIGHTLOSS
MY RATING FOR THIS JUICE RECIPE	○1 ○2 ○3 ○4 ○5 ○6 ○7 ○8 ○9 ○10

JUICE RECIPE

PREP TIME		# OF OUNCES	
JUICING TIME		# OF SERVINGS	

THIS JUICE IS FOR:

○ BREAKFAST	○ LUNCH	○ DINNER	○ HEALING

INGREDIENTS

_____
_____
_____
_____
_____
_____
_____
_____
_____
_____

HOW TO PREPARE

_____
_____
_____
_____

HOW I FELT AFTER JUICING

_____
_____

MY RESULTS	○ IMPROVED MOOD ○ IMPROVED ENERGY ○ IMPROVED FOCUS ○ WEIGHTLOSS
MY RATING FOR THIS JUICE RECIPE	○1 ○2 ○3 ○4 ○5 ○6 ○7 ○8 ○9 ○10

JUICE RECIPE

PREP TIME		# OF OUNCES	
JUICING TIME		# OF SERVINGS	

THIS JUICE IS FOR:

○ BREAKFAST	○ LUNCH	○ DINNER	○ HEALING

INGREDIENTS

_____
_____
_____
_____
_____
_____
_____
_____
_____

HOW TO PREPARE

_____
_____
_____
_____
_____

HOW I FELT AFTER JUICING

_____
_____

MY RESULTS	○ IMPROVED MOOD ○ IMPROVED ENERGY ○ IMPROVED FOCUS ○ WEIGHTLOSS
MY RATING FOR THIS JUICE RECIPE	○1 ○2 ○3 ○4 ○5 ○6 ○7 ○8 ○9 ○10

JUICE RECIPE

PREP TIME		# OF OUNCES	
JUICING TIME		# OF SERVINGS	

THIS JUICE IS FOR:

○ BREAKFAST	○ LUNCH	○ DINNER	○ HEALING

INGREDIENTS

_____

_____

_____

_____

_____

_____

_____

_____

_____

_____

HOW TO PREPARE

_____

_____

_____

_____

HOW I FELT AFTER JUICING

_____

_____

_____

MY RESULTS	○ IMPROVED MOOD ○ IMPROVED ENERGY ○ IMPROVED FOCUS ○ WEIGHTLOSS
MY RATING FOR THIS JUICE RECIPE	○ 1 ○ 2 ○ 3 ○ 4 ○ 5 ○ 6 ○ 7 ○ 8 ○ 9 ○ 10

JUICE RECIPE

PREP TIME		# OF OUNCES	
JUICING TIME		# OF SERVINGS	

THIS JUICE IS FOR:

○ BREAKFAST	○ LUNCH	○ DINNER	○ HEALING

INGREDIENTS

_____
_____
_____
_____
_____
_____
_____
_____

HOW TO PREPARE

_____
_____
_____
_____
_____

HOW I FELT AFTER JUICING

_____
_____
_____

MY RESULTS	○ IMPROVED MOOD ○ IMPROVED ENERGY ○ IMPROVED FOCUS ○ WEIGHTLOSS
MY RATING FOR THIS JUICE RECIPE	○1 ○2 ○3 ○4 ○5 ○6 ○7 ○8 ○9 ○10

JUICE RECIPE

PREP TIME		# OF OUNCES	
JUICING TIME		# OF SERVINGS	

THIS JUICE IS FOR:

○ BREAKFAST	○ LUNCH	○ DINNER	○ HEALING

INGREDIENTS

_____
_____
_____
_____
_____
_____
_____
_____
_____
_____
_____
_____

HOW TO PREPARE

_____
_____
_____
_____
_____

HOW I FELT AFTER JUICING

_____
_____
_____

MY RESULTS	○ IMPROVED MOOD ○ IMPROVED ENERGY ○ IMPROVED FOCUS ○ WEIGHTLOSS
MY RATING FOR THIS JUICE RECIPE	○1 ○2 ○3 ○4 ○5 ○6 ○7 ○8 ○9 ○10

JUICE RECIPE

PREP TIME		# OF OUNCES	
JUICING TIME		# OF SERVINGS	

THIS JUICE IS FOR:

○ BREAKFAST	○ LUNCH	○ DINNER	○ HEALING

INGREDIENTS

_____
_____
_____
_____
_____
_____
_____
_____

HOW TO PREPARE

_____
_____
_____
_____

HOW I FELT AFTER JUICING

_____
_____
_____

MY RESULTS	○ IMPROVED MOOD ○ IMPROVED ENERGY ○ IMPROVED FOCUS ○ WEIGHTLOSS
MY RATING FOR THIS JUICE RECIPE	○1 ○2 ○3 ○4 ○5 ○6 ○7 ○8 ○9 ○10

JUICE RECIPE

PREP TIME		# OF OUNCES	
JUICING TIME		# OF SERVINGS	

THIS JUICE IS FOR:

○ BREAKFAST	○ LUNCH	○ DINNER	○ HEALING

INGREDIENTS

_____
_____
_____
_____
_____
_____
_____
_____

HOW TO PREPARE

_____
_____
_____
_____

HOW I FELT AFTER JUICING

_____
_____

MY RESULTS	○ IMPROVED MOOD ○ IMPROVED ENERGY ○ IMPROVED FOCUS ○ WEIGHTLOSS
MY RATING FOR THIS JUICE RECIPE	○1 ○2 ○3 ○4 ○5 ○6 ○7 ○8 ○9 ○10

JUICE RECIPE

PREP TIME		# OF OUNCES	
JUICING TIME		# OF SERVINGS	

THIS JUICE IS FOR:

○ BREAKFAST   ○ LUNCH   ○ DINNER   ○ HEALING

INGREDIENTS

_____
_____
_____
_____
_____
_____
_____
_____
_____
_____

HOW TO PREPARE

_____
_____
_____
_____

HOW I FELT AFTER JUICING

_____
_____
_____

MY RESULTS	○ IMPROVED MOOD ○ IMPROVED ENERGY ○ IMPROVED FOCUS ○ WEIGHTLOSS
MY RATING FOR THIS JUICE RECIPE	○1 ○2 ○3 ○4 ○5 ○6 ○7 ○8 ○9 ○10

JUICE RECIPE

PREP TIME		# OF OUNCES	
JUICING TIME		# OF SERVINGS	

THIS JUICE IS FOR:

○ BREAKFAST	○ LUNCH	○ DINNER	○ HEALING

INGREDIENTS

_____
_____
_____
_____
_____
_____
_____
_____
_____
_____

HOW TO PREPARE

_____
_____
_____
_____

HOW I FELT AFTER JUICING

_____
_____

MY RESULTS	○ IMPROVED MOOD ○ IMPROVED ENERGY ○ IMPROVED FOCUS ○ WEIGHTLOSS
MY RATING FOR THIS JUICE RECIPE	○1 ○2 ○3 ○4 ○5 ○6 ○7 ○8 ○9 ○10

JUICE RECIPE

PREP TIME		# OF OUNCES	
JUICING TIME		# OF SERVINGS	

THIS JUICE IS FOR:

○ BREAKFAST   ○ LUNCH   ○ DINNER   ○ HEALING

INGREDIENTS

_____
_____
_____
_____
_____
_____
_____
_____
_____

HOW TO PREPARE

_____
_____
_____
_____

HOW I FELT AFTER JUICING

_____
_____

MY RESULTS	○ IMPROVED MOOD ○ IMPROVED ENERGY ○ IMPROVED FOCUS ○ WEIGHTLOSS
MY RATING FOR THIS JUICE RECIPE	○1 ○2 ○3 ○4 ○5 ○6 ○7 ○8 ○9 ○10

JUICE RECIPE

PREP TIME		# OF OUNCES	
JUICING TIME		# OF SERVINGS	

THIS JUICE IS FOR:

○ BREAKFAST	○ LUNCH	○ DINNER	○ HEALING

INGREDIENTS

_____
_____
_____
_____
_____
_____
_____
_____
_____
_____

HOW TO PREPARE

_____
_____
_____
_____

HOW I FELT AFTER JUICING

_____
_____

MY RESULTS	○ IMPROVED MOOD ○ IMPROVED ENERGY ○ IMPROVED FOCUS ○ WEIGHTLOSS
MY RATING FOR THIS JUICE RECIPE	○1 ○2 ○3 ○4 ○5 ○6 ○7 ○8 ○9 ○10

JUICE RECIPE

PREP TIME		# OF OUNCES	
JUICING TIME		# OF SERVINGS	

THIS JUICE IS FOR:

○ BREAKFAST	○ LUNCH	○ DINNER	○ HEALING

INGREDIENTS

_____
_____
_____
_____
_____
_____
_____
_____

HOW TO PREPARE

_____
_____
_____
_____

HOW I FELT AFTER JUICING

_____
_____

MY RESULTS	○ IMPROVED MOOD ○ IMPROVED ENERGY ○ IMPROVED FOCUS ○ WEIGHTLOSS
MY RATING FOR THIS JUICE RECIPE	○1 ○2 ○3 ○4 ○5 ○6 ○7 ○8 ○9 ○10

JUICE RECIPE

PREP TIME		# OF OUNCES	
JUICING TIME		# OF SERVINGS	

THIS JUICE IS FOR:

○ BREAKFAST	○ LUNCH	○ DINNER	○ HEALING

INGREDIENTS

_____
_____
_____
_____
_____
_____
_____
_____
_____

HOW TO PREPARE

_____
_____
_____
_____

HOW I FELT AFTER JUICING

_____
_____

MY RESULTS	○ IMPROVED MOOD ○ IMPROVED ENERGY ○ IMPROVED FOCUS ○ WEIGHTLOSS
MY RATING FOR THIS JUICE RECIPE	○1 ○2 ○3 ○4 ○5 ○6 ○7 ○8 ○9 ○10

JUICE RECIPE

PREP TIME		# OF OUNCES	
JUICING TIME		# OF SERVINGS	

THIS JUICE IS FOR:

○ BREAKFAST	○ LUNCH	○ DINNER	○ HEALING

INGREDIENTS

_____
_____
_____
_____
_____
_____
_____
_____
_____

HOW TO PREPARE

_____
_____
_____
_____
_____

HOW I FELT AFTER JUICING

_____
_____

MY RESULTS	○ IMPROVED MOOD ○ IMPROVED ENERGY ○ IMPROVED FOCUS ○ WEIGHTLOSS
MY RATING FOR THIS JUICE RECIPE	○1 ○2 ○3 ○4 ○5 ○6 ○7 ○8 ○9 ○10

JUICE RECIPE

PREP TIME		# OF OUNCES	
JUICING TIME		# OF SERVINGS	

THIS JUICE IS FOR:

○ BREAKFAST	○ LUNCH	○ DINNER	○ HEALING

INGREDIENTS

_____
_____
_____
_____
_____
_____
_____
_____
_____

HOW TO PREPARE

_____
_____
_____
_____

HOW I FELT AFTER JUICING

_____
_____

MY RESULTS	○ IMPROVED MOOD ○ IMPROVED ENERGY ○ IMPROVED FOCUS ○ WEIGHTLOSS
MY RATING FOR THIS JUICE RECIPE	○1 ○2 ○3 ○4 ○5 ○6 ○7 ○8 ○9 ○10

JUICE RECIPE

PREP TIME		# OF OUNCES	
JUICING TIME		# OF SERVINGS	

THIS JUICE IS FOR:

○ BREAKFAST   ○ LUNCH   ○ DINNER   ○ HEALING

INGREDIENTS

_____
_____
_____
_____
_____
_____
_____
_____

HOW TO PREPARE

_____
_____
_____
_____

HOW I FELT AFTER JUICING

_____
_____

MY RESULTS	○ IMPROVED MOOD ○ IMPROVED ENERGY ○ IMPROVED FOCUS ○ WEIGHTLOSS
MY RATING FOR THIS JUICE RECIPE	○1 ○2 ○3 ○4 ○5 ○6 ○7 ○8 ○9 ○10

JUICE RECIPE

PREP TIME		# OF OUNCES	
JUICING TIME		# OF SERVINGS	

THIS JUICE IS FOR:

○ BREAKFAST	○ LUNCH	○ DINNER	○ HEALING

INGREDIENTS

HOW TO PREPARE

HOW I FELT AFTER JUICING

MY RESULTS	○ IMPROVED MOOD ○ IMPROVED ENERGY ○ IMPROVED FOCUS ○ WEIGHTLOSS
MY RATING FOR THIS JUICE RECIPE	○1 ○2 ○3 ○4 ○5 ○6 ○7 ○8 ○9 ○10

JUICE RECIPE

PREP TIME		# OF OUNCES	
JUICING TIME		# OF SERVINGS	

THIS JUICE IS FOR:

○ BREAKFAST	○ LUNCH	○ DINNER	○ HEALING

INGREDIENTS

_____
_____
_____
_____
_____
_____
_____
_____

HOW TO PREPARE

_____
_____
_____
_____

HOW I FELT AFTER JUICING

_____
_____
_____

MY RESULTS	○ IMPROVED MOOD ○ IMPROVED ENERGY ○ IMPROVED FOCUS ○ WEIGHTLOSS
MY RATING FOR THIS JUICE RECIPE	○ 1 ○ 2 ○ 3 ○ 4 ○ 5 ○ 6 ○ 7 ○ 8 ○ 9 ○ 10

JUICE RECIPE

PREP TIME		# OF OUNCES	
JUICING TIME		# OF SERVINGS	

THIS JUICE IS FOR:

○ BREAKFAST	○ LUNCH	○ DINNER	○ HEALING

INGREDIENTS

_____
_____
_____
_____
_____
_____
_____
_____
_____
_____

HOW TO PREPARE

_____
_____
_____

HOW I FELT AFTER JUICING

_____
_____

MY RESULTS	○ IMPROVED MOOD ○ IMPROVED ENERGY ○ IMPROVED FOCUS ○ WEIGHTLOSS
MY RATING FOR THIS JUICE RECIPE	○1 ○2 ○3 ○4 ○5 ○6 ○7 ○8 ○9 ○10

JUICE RECIPE

PREP TIME		# OF OUNCES	
JUICING TIME		# OF SERVINGS	

THIS JUICE IS FOR:

○ BREAKFAST   ○ LUNCH   ○ DINNER   ○ HEALING

INGREDIENTS

_____
_____
_____
_____
_____
_____
_____
_____
_____

HOW TO PREPARE

_____
_____
_____
_____

HOW I FELT AFTER JUICING

_____
_____

MY RESULTS	○ IMPROVED MOOD ○ IMPROVED ENERGY ○ IMPROVED FOCUS ○ WEIGHTLOSS
MY RATING FOR THIS JUICE RECIPE	○1 ○2 ○3 ○4 ○5 ○6 ○7 ○8 ○9 ○10

JUICE RECIPE

PREP TIME		# OF OUNCES	
JUICING TIME		# OF SERVINGS	

THIS JUICE IS FOR:

○ BREAKFAST	○ LUNCH	○ DINNER	○ HEALING

INGREDIENTS

_____
_____
_____
_____
_____
_____
_____
_____
_____

HOW TO PREPARE

_____
_____
_____
_____

HOW I FELT AFTER JUICING

_____
_____

MY RESULTS	○ IMPROVED MOOD ○ IMPROVED ENERGY ○ IMPROVED FOCUS ○ WEIGHTLOSS
MY RATING FOR THIS JUICE RECIPE	○1 ○2 ○3 ○4 ○5 ○6 ○7 ○8 ○9 ○10

JUICE RECIPE

PREP TIME		# OF OUNCES	
JUICING TIME		# OF SERVINGS	

THIS JUICE IS FOR:

○ BREAKFAST	○ LUNCH	○ DINNER	○ HEALING

INGREDIENTS

_____

_____

_____

_____

_____

_____

_____

_____

HOW TO PREPARE

_____

_____

_____

_____

HOW I FELT AFTER JUICING

_____

_____

_____

MY RESULTS	○ IMPROVED MOOD ○ IMPROVED ENERGY ○ IMPROVED FOCUS ○ WEIGHTLOSS
MY RATING FOR THIS JUICE RECIPE	○1 ○2 ○3 ○4 ○5 ○6 ○7 ○8 ○9 ○10

JUICE RECIPE

PREP TIME		# OF OUNCES	
JUICING TIME		# OF SERVINGS	

THIS JUICE IS FOR:

○ BREAKFAST	○ LUNCH	○ DINNER	○ HEALING

INGREDIENTS

HOW TO PREPARE

HOW I FELT AFTER JUICING

MY RESULTS	○ IMPROVED MOOD ○ IMPROVED ENERGY ○ IMPROVED FOCUS ○ WEIGHTLOSS
MY RATING FOR THIS JUICE RECIPE	○1 ○2 ○3 ○4 ○5 ○6 ○7 ○8 ○9 ○10

JUICE RECIPE

PREP TIME		# OF OUNCES	
JUICING TIME		# OF SERVINGS	

THIS JUICE IS FOR:

○ BREAKFAST	○ LUNCH	○ DINNER	○ HEALING

INGREDIENTS

_____

_____

_____

_____

_____

_____

_____

_____

HOW TO PREPARE

_____

_____

_____

_____

HOW I FELT AFTER JUICING

_____

_____

_____

MY RESULTS	○ IMPROVED MOOD ○ IMPROVED ENERGY ○ IMPROVED FOCUS ○ WEIGHTLOSS
MY RATING FOR THIS JUICE RECIPE	○1 ○2 ○3 ○4 ○5 ○6 ○7 ○8 ○9 ○10

JUICE RECIPE

PREP TIME		# OF OUNCES	
JUICING TIME		# OF SERVINGS	

THIS JUICE IS FOR:

○ BREAKFAST   ○ LUNCH   ○ DINNER   ○ HEALING

INGREDIENTS

_____
_____
_____
_____
_____
_____
_____
_____
_____
_____

HOW TO PREPARE

_____
_____
_____
_____

HOW I FELT AFTER JUICING

_____
_____

MY RESULTS	○ IMPROVED MOOD ○ IMPROVED ENERGY ○ IMPROVED FOCUS ○ WEIGHTLOSS
MY RATING FOR THIS JUICE RECIPE	○1 ○2 ○3 ○4 ○5 ○6 ○7 ○8 ○9 ○10

JUICE RECIPE

PREP TIME		# OF OUNCES	
JUICING TIME		# OF SERVINGS	

THIS JUICE IS FOR:

○ BREAKFAST	○ LUNCH	○ DINNER	○ HEALING

INGREDIENTS

_____
_____
_____
_____
_____
_____
_____
_____
_____
_____

HOW TO PREPARE

_____
_____
_____
_____

HOW I FELT AFTER JUICING

_____
_____
_____

MY RESULTS	○ IMPROVED MOOD ○ IMPROVED ENERGY ○ IMPROVED FOCUS ○ WEIGHTLOSS
MY RATING FOR THIS JUICE RECIPE	○1 ○2 ○3 ○4 ○5 ○6 ○7 ○8 ○9 ○10

JUICE RECIPE

PREP TIME		# OF OUNCES	
JUICING TIME		# OF SERVINGS	

THIS JUICE IS FOR:

○ BREAKFAST   ○ LUNCH   ○ DINNER   ○ HEALING

INGREDIENTS

_____
_____
_____
_____
_____
_____
_____
_____
_____
_____

HOW TO PREPARE

_____
_____
_____
_____

HOW I FELT AFTER JUICING

_____
_____

MY RESULTS	○ IMPROVED MOOD ○ IMPROVED ENERGY ○ IMPROVED FOCUS ○ WEIGHTLOSS
MY RATING FOR THIS JUICE RECIPE	○1 ○2 ○3 ○4 ○5 ○6 ○7 ○8 ○9 ○10

JUICE RECIPE

PREP TIME		# OF OUNCES	
JUICING TIME		# OF SERVINGS	

THIS JUICE IS FOR:

○ BREAKFAST   ○ LUNCH   ○ DINNER   ○ HEALING

INGREDIENTS

_____
_____
_____
_____
_____
_____
_____
_____
_____

HOW TO PREPARE

_____
_____
_____
_____

HOW I FELT AFTER JUICING

_____
_____

MY RESULTS	○ IMPROVED MOOD ○ IMPROVED ENERGY ○ IMPROVED FOCUS ○ WEIGHTLOSS
MY RATING FOR THIS JUICE RECIPE	○1 ○2 ○3 ○4 ○5 ○6 ○7 ○8 ○9 ○10

JUICE RECIPE

PREP TIME		# OF OUNCES	
JUICING TIME		# OF SERVINGS	

THIS JUICE IS FOR:

○ BREAKFAST	○ LUNCH	○ DINNER	○ HEALING

INGREDIENTS

HOW TO PREPARE

HOW I FELT AFTER JUICING

MY RESULTS	○ IMPROVED MOOD ○ IMPROVED ENERGY ○ IMPROVED FOCUS ○ WEIGHTLOSS
MY RATING FOR THIS JUICE RECIPE	○ 1 ○ 2 ○ 3 ○ 4 ○ 5 ○ 6 ○ 7 ○ 8 ○ 9 ○ 10

JUICE RECIPE

PREP TIME		# OF OUNCES	
JUICING TIME		# OF SERVINGS	

THIS JUICE IS FOR:

○ BREAKFAST	○ LUNCH	○ DINNER	○ HEALING

INGREDIENTS

_____
_____
_____
_____
_____
_____
_____
_____

HOW TO PREPARE

_____
_____
_____
_____

HOW I FELT AFTER JUICING

_____
_____
_____

MY RESULTS	○ IMPROVED MOOD ○ IMPROVED ENERGY ○ IMPROVED FOCUS ○ WEIGHTLOSS
MY RATING FOR THIS JUICE RECIPE	○1 ○2 ○3 ○4 ○5 ○6 ○7 ○8 ○9 ○10

JUICE RECIPE

PREP TIME		# OF OUNCES	
JUICING TIME		# OF SERVINGS	

THIS JUICE IS FOR:

○ BREAKFAST	○ LUNCH	○ DINNER	○ HEALING

INGREDIENTS

_____

_____

_____

_____

_____

_____

_____

_____

_____

HOW TO PREPARE

_____

_____

_____

_____

HOW I FELT AFTER JUICING

_____

_____

MY RESULTS	○ IMPROVED MOOD ○ IMPROVED ENERGY ○ IMPROVED FOCUS ○ WEIGHTLOSS
MY RATING FOR THIS JUICE RECIPE	○1 ○2 ○3 ○4 ○5 ○6 ○7 ○8 ○9 ○10

JUICE RECIPE

PREP TIME		# OF OUNCES	
JUICING TIME		# OF SERVINGS	

THIS JUICE IS FOR:

○ BREAKFAST ○ LUNCH ○ DINNER ○ HEALING

INGREDIENTS

_____
_____
_____
_____
_____
_____
_____
_____

HOW TO PREPARE

_____
_____
_____
_____

HOW I FELT AFTER JUICING

_____
_____
_____

MY RESULTS	○ IMPROVED MOOD ○ IMPROVED ENERGY ○ IMPROVED FOCUS ○ WEIGHTLOSS
MY RATING FOR THIS JUICE RECIPE	○1 ○2 ○3 ○4 ○5 ○6 ○7 ○8 ○9 ○10

JUICE RECIPE

PREP TIME		# OF OUNCES	
JUICING TIME		# OF SERVINGS	

THIS JUICE IS FOR:

○ BREAKFAST ○ LUNCH ○ DINNER ○ HEALING

INGREDIENTS

_____
_____
_____
_____
_____
_____
_____
_____
_____
_____

HOW TO PREPARE

_____
_____
_____
_____

HOW I FELT AFTER JUICING

_____
_____
_____

MY RESULTS	○ IMPROVED MOOD ○ IMPROVED ENERGY ○ IMPROVED FOCUS ○ WEIGHTLOSS
MY RATING FOR THIS JUICE RECIPE	○1 ○2 ○3 ○4 ○5 ○6 ○7 ○8 ○9 ○10

JUICE RECIPE

PREP TIME		# OF OUNCES	
JUICING TIME		# OF SERVINGS	

THIS JUICE IS FOR:

○ BREAKFAST ○ LUNCH ○ DINNER ○ HEALING

INGREDIENTS

HOW TO PREPARE

HOW I FELT AFTER JUICING

MY RESULTS	○ IMPROVED MOOD ○ IMPROVED ENERGY ○ IMPROVED FOCUS ○ WEIGHTLOSS
MY RATING FOR THIS JUICE RECIPE	○1 ○2 ○3 ○4 ○5 ○6 ○7 ○8 ○9 ○10

JUICE RECIPE

PREP TIME		# OF OUNCES	
JUICING TIME		# OF SERVINGS	

THIS JUICE IS FOR:

| ○ BREAKFAST | ○ LUNCH | ○ DINNER | ○ HEALING |

INGREDIENTS

HOW TO PREPARE

HOW I FELT AFTER JUICING

MY RESULTS	○ IMPROVED MOOD ○ IMPROVED ENERGY ○ IMPROVED FOCUS ○ WEIGHTLOSS
MY RATING FOR THIS JUICE RECIPE	○1 ○2 ○3 ○4 ○5 ○6 ○7 ○8 ○9 ○10

JUICE RECIPE

PREP TIME		# OF OUNCES	
JUICING TIME		# OF SERVINGS	

THIS JUICE IS FOR:

○ BREAKFAST   ○ LUNCH   ○ DINNER   ○ HEALING

INGREDIENTS

_____
_____
_____
_____
_____
_____
_____

HOW TO PREPARE

_____
_____
_____
_____

HOW I FELT AFTER JUICING

_____
_____

MY RESULTS	○ IMPROVED MOOD ○ IMPROVED ENERGY ○ IMPROVED FOCUS ○ WEIGHTLOSS
MY RATING FOR THIS JUICE RECIPE	○1 ○2 ○3 ○4 ○5 ○6 ○7 ○8 ○9 ○10

JUICE RECIPE

PREP TIME		# OF OUNCES	
JUICING TIME		# OF SERVINGS	

THIS JUICE IS FOR:

○ BREAKFAST	○ LUNCH	○ DINNER	○ HEALING

INGREDIENTS

_____
_____
_____
_____
_____
_____
_____
_____
_____
_____

HOW TO PREPARE

_____
_____
_____
_____

HOW I FELT AFTER JUICING

_____
_____

MY RESULTS	○ IMPROVED MOOD ○ IMPROVED ENERGY ○ IMPROVED FOCUS ○ WEIGHTLOSS
MY RATING FOR THIS JUICE RECIPE	○1 ○2 ○3 ○4 ○5 ○6 ○7 ○8 ○9 ○10

JUICE RECIPE

PREP TIME		# OF OUNCES	
JUICING TIME		# OF SERVINGS	

THIS JUICE IS FOR:

○ BREAKFAST   ○ LUNCH   ○ DINNER   ○ HEALING

INGREDIENTS

_____
_____
_____
_____
_____
_____
_____
_____
_____
_____

HOW TO PREPARE

_____
_____
_____
_____

HOW I FELT AFTER JUICING

_____
_____

MY RESULTS	○ IMPROVED MOOD ○ IMPROVED ENERGY ○ IMPROVED FOCUS ○ WEIGHTLOSS
MY RATING FOR THIS JUICE RECIPE	○1 ○2 ○3 ○4 ○5 ○6 ○7 ○8 ○9 ○10

JUICE RECIPE

PREP TIME		# OF OUNCES	
JUICING TIME		# OF SERVINGS	

THIS JUICE IS FOR:

○ BREAKFAST   ○ LUNCH   ○ DINNER   ○ HEALING

INGREDIENTS

_____
_____
_____
_____
_____
_____
_____
_____
_____

HOW TO PREPARE

_____
_____
_____
_____

HOW I FELT AFTER JUICING

_____
_____

MY RESULTS	○ IMPROVED MOOD ○ IMPROVED ENERGY ○ IMPROVED FOCUS ○ WEIGHTLOSS
MY RATING FOR THIS JUICE RECIPE	○1 ○2 ○3 ○4 ○5 ○6 ○7 ○8 ○9 ○10

JUICE RECIPE

PREP TIME		# OF OUNCES	
JUICING TIME		# OF SERVINGS	

THIS JUICE IS FOR:

○ BREAKFAST	○ LUNCH	○ DINNER	○ HEALING

INGREDIENTS

HOW TO PREPARE

HOW I FELT AFTER JUICING

MY RESULTS	○ IMPROVED MOOD ○ IMPROVED ENERGY ○ IMPROVED FOCUS ○ WEIGHTLOSS
MY RATING FOR THIS JUICE RECIPE	○1 ○2 ○3 ○4 ○5 ○6 ○7 ○8 ○9 ○10

JUICE RECIPE

PREP TIME		# OF OUNCES	
JUICING TIME		# OF SERVINGS	

THIS JUICE IS FOR:

○ BREAKFAST ○ LUNCH ○ DINNER ○ HEALING

INGREDIENTS

_____
_____
_____
_____
_____
_____
_____
_____
_____
_____

HOW TO PREPARE

_____
_____
_____
_____
_____

HOW I FELT AFTER JUICING

_____
_____

MY RESULTS	○ IMPROVED MOOD ○ IMPROVED ENERGY ○ IMPROVED FOCUS ○ WEIGHTLOSS
MY RATING FOR THIS JUICE RECIPE	○1 ○2 ○3 ○4 ○5 ○6 ○7 ○8 ○9 ○10

JUICE RECIPE

PREP TIME		# OF OUNCES	
JUICING TIME		# OF SERVINGS	

THIS JUICE IS FOR:

○ BREAKFAST	○ LUNCH	○ DINNER	○ HEALING

INGREDIENTS

_____

_____

_____

_____

_____

_____

_____

_____

HOW TO PREPARE

_____

_____

_____

_____

HOW I FELT AFTER JUICING

_____

_____

_____

MY RESULTS	○ IMPROVED MOOD ○ IMPROVED ENERGY ○ IMPROVED FOCUS ○ WEIGHTLOSS
MY RATING FOR THIS JUICE RECIPE	○1 ○2 ○3 ○4 ○5 ○6 ○7 ○8 ○9 ○10

JUICE RECIPE

PREP TIME		# OF OUNCES	
JUICING TIME		# OF SERVINGS	

THIS JUICE IS FOR:

○ BREAKFAST	○ LUNCH	○ DINNER	○ HEALING

INGREDIENTS

_____
_____
_____
_____
_____
_____
_____
_____
_____

HOW TO PREPARE

_____
_____
_____
_____
_____

HOW I FELT AFTER JUICING

_____
_____

MY RESULTS	○ IMPROVED MOOD ○ IMPROVED ENERGY ○ IMPROVED FOCUS ○ WEIGHTLOSS
MY RATING FOR THIS JUICE RECIPE	○ 1 ○ 2 ○ 3 ○ 4 ○ 5 ○ 6 ○ 7 ○ 8 ○ 9 ○ 10

JUICE RECIPE

PREP TIME		# OF OUNCES	
JUICING TIME		# OF SERVINGS	

THIS JUICE IS FOR:

○ BREAKFAST ○ LUNCH ○ DINNER ○ HEALING

INGREDIENTS

_____
_____
_____
_____
_____
_____
_____
_____
_____

HOW TO PREPARE

_____
_____
_____
_____
_____

HOW I FELT AFTER JUICING

_____
_____

MY RESULTS	○ IMPROVED MOOD ○ IMPROVED ENERGY ○ IMPROVED FOCUS ○ WEIGHTLOSS
MY RATING FOR THIS JUICE RECIPE	○1 ○2 ○3 ○4 ○5 ○6 ○7 ○8 ○9 ○10

JUICE RECIPE

PREP TIME		# OF OUNCES	
JUICING TIME		# OF SERVINGS	

THIS JUICE IS FOR:

| ○ BREAKFAST | ○ LUNCH | ○ DINNER | ○ HEALING |

INGREDIENTS

_____
_____
_____
_____
_____
_____
_____
_____
_____

HOW TO PREPARE

_____
_____
_____
_____

HOW I FELT AFTER JUICING

_____
_____

MY RESULTS	○ IMPROVED MOOD ○ IMPROVED ENERGY ○ IMPROVED FOCUS ○ WEIGHTLOSS
MY RATING FOR THIS JUICE RECIPE	○1 ○2 ○3 ○4 ○5 ○6 ○7 ○8 ○9 ○10

JUICE RECIPE

PREP TIME		# OF OUNCES	
JUICING TIME		# OF SERVINGS	

THIS JUICE IS FOR:			
○ BREAKFAST	○ LUNCH	○ DINNER	○ HEALING

INGREDIENTS

_____
_____
_____
_____
_____
_____
_____
_____

HOW TO PREPARE

_____
_____
_____
_____

HOW I FELT AFTER JUICING

_____
_____

MY RESULTS	○ IMPROVED MOOD ○ IMPROVED ENERGY ○ IMPROVED FOCUS ○ WEIGHTLOSS
MY RATING FOR THIS JUICE RECIPE	○1 ○2 ○3 ○4 ○5 ○6 ○7 ○8 ○9 ○10

JUICE RECIPE

PREP TIME		# OF OUNCES	
JUICING TIME		# OF SERVINGS	

THIS JUICE IS FOR:

○ BREAKFAST	○ LUNCH	○ DINNER	○ HEALING

INGREDIENTS

HOW TO PREPARE

HOW I FELT AFTER JUICING

MY RESULTS	○ IMPROVED MOOD ○ IMPROVED ENERGY ○ IMPROVED FOCUS ○ WEIGHTLOSS
MY RATING FOR THIS JUICE RECIPE	○ 1 ○ 2 ○ 3 ○ 4 ○ 5 ○ 6 ○ 7 ○ 8 ○ 9 ○ 10

JUICE RECIPE

PREP TIME		# OF OUNCES	
JUICING TIME		# OF SERVINGS	

THIS JUICE IS FOR:			
○ BREAKFAST	○ LUNCH	○ DINNER	○ HEALING

INGREDIENTS

_____

_____

_____

_____

_____

_____

_____

_____

HOW TO PREPARE

_____

_____

_____

_____

HOW I FELT AFTER JUICING

_____

_____

_____

MY RESULTS	○ IMPROVED MOOD ○ IMPROVED ENERGY ○ IMPROVED FOCUS ○ WEIGHTLOSS
MY RATING FOR THIS JUICE RECIPE	○1 ○2 ○3 ○4 ○5 ○6 ○7 ○8 ○9 ○10

JUICE RECIPE

PREP TIME		# OF OUNCES	
JUICING TIME		# OF SERVINGS	

THIS JUICE IS FOR:

○ BREAKFAST ○ LUNCH ○ DINNER ○ HEALING

INGREDIENTS

HOW TO PREPARE

HOW I FELT AFTER JUICING

MY RESULTS	○ IMPROVED MOOD ○ IMPROVED ENERGY ○ IMPROVED FOCUS ○ WEIGHTLOSS
MY RATING FOR THIS JUICE RECIPE	○1 ○2 ○3 ○4 ○5 ○6 ○7 ○8 ○9 ○10

JUICE RECIPE

PREP TIME		# OF OUNCES	
JUICING TIME		# OF SERVINGS	

THIS JUICE IS FOR:

○ BREAKFAST   ○ LUNCH   ○ DINNER   ○ HEALING

INGREDIENTS

_____
_____
_____
_____
_____
_____
_____
_____
_____
_____

HOW TO PREPARE

_____
_____
_____
_____
_____

HOW I FELT AFTER JUICING

_____
_____
_____

MY RESULTS	○ IMPROVED MOOD ○ IMPROVED ENERGY ○ IMPROVED FOCUS ○ WEIGHTLOSS
MY RATING FOR THIS JUICE RECIPE	○1 ○2 ○3 ○4 ○5 ○6 ○7 ○8 ○9 ○10

JUICE RECIPE

PREP TIME		# OF OUNCES	
JUICING TIME		# OF SERVINGS	

THIS JUICE IS FOR:

○ BREAKFAST	○ LUNCH	○ DINNER	○ HEALING

INGREDIENTS

_____
_____
_____
_____
_____
_____
_____
_____
_____
_____

HOW TO PREPARE

_____
_____
_____
_____

HOW I FELT AFTER JUICING

_____
_____

MY RESULTS	○ IMPROVED MOOD ○ IMPROVED ENERGY ○ IMPROVED FOCUS ○ WEIGHTLOSS
MY RATING FOR THIS JUICE RECIPE	○1 ○2 ○3 ○4 ○5 ○6 ○7 ○8 ○9 ○10

JUICE RECIPE

PREP TIME		# OF OUNCES	
JUICING TIME		# OF SERVINGS	

THIS JUICE IS FOR:

○ BREAKFAST	○ LUNCH	○ DINNER	○ HEALING

INGREDIENTS

_____
_____
_____
_____
_____
_____
_____
_____

HOW TO PREPARE

_____
_____
_____
_____

HOW I FELT AFTER JUICING

_____
_____
_____

MY RESULTS	○ IMPROVED MOOD ○ IMPROVED ENERGY ○ IMPROVED FOCUS ○ WEIGHTLOSS
MY RATING FOR THIS JUICE RECIPE	○1 ○2 ○3 ○4 ○5 ○6 ○7 ○8 ○9 ○10

JUICE RECIPE

PREP TIME		# OF OUNCES	
JUICING TIME		# OF SERVINGS	

THIS JUICE IS FOR:

○ BREAKFAST	○ LUNCH	○ DINNER	○ HEALING

INGREDIENTS

_____
_____
_____
_____
_____
_____
_____
_____
_____
_____

HOW TO PREPARE

_____
_____
_____
_____

HOW I FELT AFTER JUICING

_____
_____

MY RESULTS	○ IMPROVED MOOD ○ IMPROVED ENERGY ○ IMPROVED FOCUS ○ WEIGHTLOSS
MY RATING FOR THIS JUICE RECIPE	○1 ○2 ○3 ○4 ○5 ○6 ○7 ○8 ○9 ○10

JUICE RECIPE

PREP TIME		# OF OUNCES	
JUICING TIME		# OF SERVINGS	

THIS JUICE IS FOR:

○ BREAKFAST	○ LUNCH	○ DINNER	○ HEALING

INGREDIENTS

_____
_____
_____
_____
_____
_____
_____
_____

HOW TO PREPARE

_____
_____
_____
_____

HOW I FELT AFTER JUICING

_____
_____

MY RESULTS	○ IMPROVED MOOD ○ IMPROVED ENERGY ○ IMPROVED FOCUS ○ WEIGHTLOSS
MY RATING FOR THIS JUICE RECIPE	○1 ○2 ○3 ○4 ○5 ○6 ○7 ○8 ○9 ○10

JUICE RECIPE

PREP TIME		# OF OUNCES	
JUICING TIME		# OF SERVINGS	

THIS JUICE IS FOR:

○ BREAKFAST	○ LUNCH	○ DINNER	○ HEALING

INGREDIENTS

_____
_____
_____
_____
_____
_____
_____
_____

HOW TO PREPARE

_____
_____
_____
_____

HOW I FELT AFTER JUICING

_____
_____

MY RESULTS	○ IMPROVED MOOD ○ IMPROVED ENERGY ○ IMPROVED FOCUS ○ WEIGHTLOSS
MY RATING FOR THIS JUICE RECIPE	○1 ○2 ○3 ○4 ○5 ○6 ○7 ○8 ○9 ○10

JUICE RECIPE

PREP TIME		# OF OUNCES	
JUICING TIME		# OF SERVINGS	

THIS JUICE IS FOR:

○ BREAKFAST   ○ LUNCH   ○ DINNER   ○ HEALING

INGREDIENTS

_____
_____
_____
_____
_____
_____
_____
_____
_____
_____

HOW TO PREPARE

_____
_____
_____
_____
_____

HOW I FELT AFTER JUICING

_____
_____
_____

MY RESULTS	○ IMPROVED MOOD ○ IMPROVED ENERGY ○ IMPROVED FOCUS ○ WEIGHTLOSS
MY RATING FOR THIS JUICE RECIPE	○1 ○2 ○3 ○4 ○5 ○6 ○7 ○8 ○9 ○10

JUICE RECIPE

PREP TIME		# OF OUNCES	
JUICING TIME		# OF SERVINGS	

THIS JUICE IS FOR:

○ BREAKFAST ○ LUNCH ○ DINNER ○ HEALING

INGREDIENTS

_____
_____
_____
_____
_____
_____
_____
_____
_____
_____

HOW TO PREPARE

_____
_____
_____
_____
_____

HOW I FELT AFTER JUICING

_____
_____

MY RESULTS	○ IMPROVED MOOD ○ IMPROVED ENERGY ○ IMPROVED FOCUS ○ WEIGHTLOSS
MY RATING FOR THIS JUICE RECIPE	○1 ○2 ○3 ○4 ○5 ○6 ○7 ○8 ○9 ○10

JUICE RECIPE

PREP TIME		# OF OUNCES	
JUICING TIME		# OF SERVINGS	

THIS JUICE IS FOR:

○ BREAKFAST	○ LUNCH	○ DINNER	○ HEALING

INGREDIENTS

_____
_____
_____
_____
_____
_____
_____
_____
_____

HOW TO PREPARE

_____
_____
_____
_____

HOW I FELT AFTER JUICING

_____
_____

MY RESULTS	○ IMPROVED MOOD ○ IMPROVED ENERGY ○ IMPROVED FOCUS ○ WEIGHTLOSS
MY RATING FOR THIS JUICE RECIPE	○1 ○2 ○3 ○4 ○5 ○6 ○7 ○8 ○9 ○10

JUICE RECIPE

PREP TIME		# OF OUNCES	
JUICING TIME		# OF SERVINGS	

THIS JUICE IS FOR:

○ BREAKFAST ○ LUNCH ○ DINNER ○ HEALING

INGREDIENTS

HOW TO PREPARE

HOW I FELT AFTER JUICING

MY RESULTS	○ IMPROVED MOOD ○ IMPROVED ENERGY ○ IMPROVED FOCUS ○ WEIGHTLOSS
MY RATING FOR THIS JUICE RECIPE	○1 ○2 ○3 ○4 ○5 ○6 ○7 ○8 ○9 ○10

JUICE RECIPE

PREP TIME		# OF OUNCES	
JUICING TIME		# OF SERVINGS	

THIS JUICE IS FOR:

○ BREAKFAST   ○ LUNCH   ○ DINNER   ○ HEALING

INGREDIENTS

_____
_____
_____
_____
_____
_____
_____
_____
_____

HOW TO PREPARE

_____
_____
_____
_____

HOW I FELT AFTER JUICING

_____
_____

MY RESULTS	○ IMPROVED MOOD ○ IMPROVED ENERGY ○ IMPROVED FOCUS ○ WEIGHTLOSS
MY RATING FOR THIS JUICE RECIPE	○ 1 ○ 2 ○ 3 ○ 4 ○ 5 ○ 6 ○ 7 ○ 8 ○ 9 ○ 10

JUICE RECIPE

PREP TIME		# OF OUNCES	
JUICING TIME		# OF SERVINGS	

THIS JUICE IS FOR:

○ BREAKFAST   ○ LUNCH   ○ DINNER   ○ HEALING

INGREDIENTS

_____
_____
_____
_____
_____
_____
_____
_____

HOW TO PREPARE

_____
_____
_____
_____

HOW I FELT AFTER JUICING

_____
_____

MY RESULTS	○ IMPROVED MOOD ○ IMPROVED ENERGY ○ IMPROVED FOCUS ○ WEIGHTLOSS
MY RATING FOR THIS JUICE RECIPE	○1 ○2 ○3 ○4 ○5 ○6 ○7 ○8 ○9 ○10

JUICE RECIPE

PREP TIME		# OF OUNCES	
JUICING TIME		# OF SERVINGS	

THIS JUICE IS FOR:

○ BREAKFAST   ○ LUNCH   ○ DINNER   ○ HEALING

INGREDIENTS

_____
_____
_____
_____
_____
_____
_____
_____
_____

HOW TO PREPARE

_____
_____
_____
_____

HOW I FELT AFTER JUICING

_____
_____

MY RESULTS	○ IMPROVED MOOD ○ IMPROVED ENERGY ○ IMPROVED FOCUS ○ WEIGHTLOSS
MY RATING FOR THIS JUICE RECIPE	○1 ○2 ○3 ○4 ○5 ○6 ○7 ○8 ○9 ○10

JUICE RECIPE

PREP TIME		# OF OUNCES	
JUICING TIME		# OF SERVINGS	

THIS JUICE IS FOR:

○ BREAKFAST ○ LUNCH ○ DINNER ○ HEALING

INGREDIENTS

_____
_____
_____
_____
_____
_____
_____
_____
_____
_____

HOW TO PREPARE

_____
_____
_____
_____

HOW I FELT AFTER JUICING

_____
_____

MY RESULTS	○ IMPROVED MOOD ○ IMPROVED ENERGY ○ IMPROVED FOCUS ○ WEIGHTLOSS
MY RATING FOR THIS JUICE RECIPE	○1 ○2 ○3 ○4 ○5 ○6 ○7 ○8 ○9 ○10

JUICE RECIPE

PREP TIME		# OF OUNCES	
JUICING TIME		# OF SERVINGS	

THIS JUICE IS FOR:

○ BREAKFAST ○ LUNCH ○ DINNER ○ HEALING

INGREDIENTS

_____
_____
_____
_____
_____
_____
_____
_____
_____

HOW TO PREPARE

_____
_____
_____
_____

HOW I FELT AFTER JUICING

_____
_____

MY RESULTS	○ IMPROVED MOOD ○ IMPROVED ENERGY ○ IMPROVED FOCUS ○ WEIGHTLOSS
MY RATING FOR THIS JUICE RECIPE	○1 ○2 ○3 ○4 ○5 ○6 ○7 ○8 ○9 ○10

JUICE RECIPE

PREP TIME		# OF OUNCES	
JUICING TIME		# OF SERVINGS	

THIS JUICE IS FOR:

○ BREAKFAST   ○ LUNCH   ○ DINNER   ○ HEALING

INGREDIENTS

___

HOW TO PREPARE

___

HOW I FELT AFTER JUICING

___

MY RESULTS	○ IMPROVED MOOD ○ IMPROVED ENERGY ○ IMPROVED FOCUS ○ WEIGHTLOSS
MY RATING FOR THIS JUICE RECIPE	○1 ○2 ○3 ○4 ○5 ○6 ○7 ○8 ○9 ○10

JUICE RECIPE

PREP TIME		# OF OUNCES	
JUICING TIME		# OF SERVINGS	

THIS JUICE IS FOR:

○ BREAKFAST　　○ LUNCH　　○ DINNER　　○ HEALING

INGREDIENTS

___

HOW TO PREPARE

___

HOW I FELT AFTER JUICING

___

MY RESULTS	○ IMPROVED MOOD　○ IMPROVED ENERGY　○ IMPROVED FOCUS　○ WEIGHTLOSS
MY RATING FOR THIS JUICE RECIPE	○1　○2　○3　○4　○5　○6　○7　○8　○9　○10

www.ingramcontent.com/pod-product-compliance
Lightning Source LLC
Chambersburg PA
CBHW052207090526
44583CB00017BA/2415